The Ultimate Air Fryer Recipe Book

Super simple, easy and delicious meat and fish

Brian Barbera

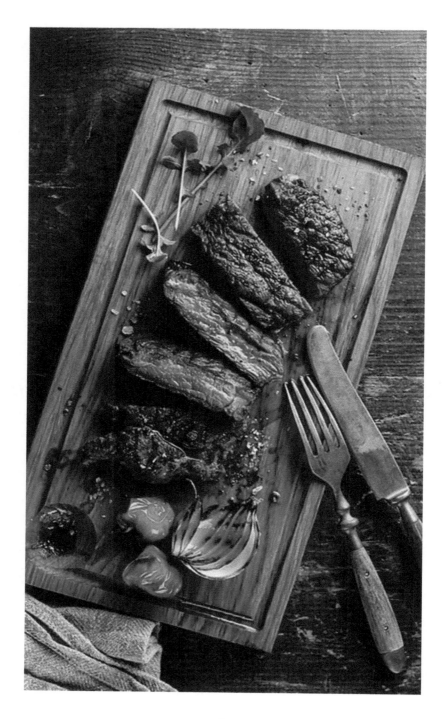

by reading this document, the reader agrees that under no circumstances is the author responsible for any losses, direct or indirect, which are incurred as a result of the use of information contained within this document, including, but not limited to, — errors, omissions, or inaccuracies.

Table of Contents

MEAT

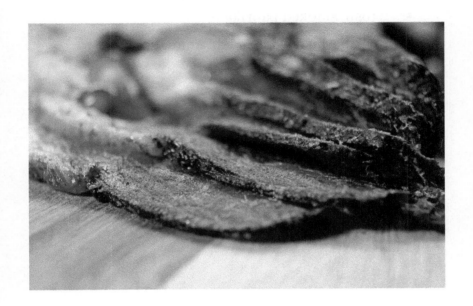

Sweet & Spicy Country-Style Ribs

Preparation Time: 10 minutes

Cooking Time: 25 minutes

Servings: 4

Ingredients:

- 2 tbsp. brown sugar
- 2 tbsp. smoked paprika
- 1 tsp. garlic powder, 1 tsp. onion powder
- 1 tsp. dry mustard
- 1 tsp. ground cumin
- 1 tsp. kosher salt, 1 tsp. black pepper
- ¼ to ½ tsp. cayenne pepper
- 1½ lb. boneless country-style pork ribs
- 1 cup barbecue sauce

Directions:

1. In a small bowl, stir together the brown sugar, paprika, garlic powder, onion powder, dry mustard, cumin, salt, black pepper, and cayenne. Mix until well combined.
2. Pat the ribs dry with a paper towel. Generously sprinkle the rub evenly over both sides of the ribs and rub in with your fingers.
3. Place the ribs in the Air Fryer basket. Set the Air Fryer to 350°F for 15 minutes. Turn the ribs and

brush with ½ cup of the barbecue sauce. Cook for an additional 10 minutes. Use a meat thermometer to ensure the pork has reached an internal temperature of 145°F. Serve with remaining barbecue sauce.

Nutrition

Calories 416, Fat 12.19g, Protein 38.39g, Carbs 36.79g

Pork Tenders with Bell Peppers

Preparation Time: 5 minutes

Cooking Time: 15 minutes

Servings: 4

Ingredients:

- 11 Oz Pork Tenderloin
- 1 Bell Pepper, in thin strips
- 1 Red Onion, sliced
- 2 Tsps. Provencal Herbs
- Black Pepper to taste
- 1 tbsp. Olive Oil
- 1/2 tbsp. Mustard

Directions:

1. Preheat the Air Fryer to 390°F.
2. In the oven dish, mix the bell pepper strips with the onion, herbs, and some salt and pepper to taste.
3. Add half a tbsp. of olive oil to the mixture

4. Cut the pork tenderloin into four pieces and rub with salt, pepper and mustard.
5. Thinly coat the pieces with remaining olive oil and place them upright in the oven dish on top of the pepper mixture
6. Place the bowl into the Air Fryer. Set the timer to 15 minutes and roast the meat and the vegetables
7. Turn the meat and mix the peppers halfway through. Serve with a fresh salad

Nutrition:

Calories 220, Fat 12.36g, Protein 23.79g, Carbs 2.45g

Wonton Meatballs

Preparation Time: 15 minutes

Cooking Time: 10 minutes

Servings: 4

Ingredients:

- 1-lb. ground pork
- 2 large eggs
- ¼ cup chopped green onions (white and green parts)
- ¼ cup chopped fresh cilantro or parsley
- 1 tbsp. minced fresh ginger
- 3 cloves garlic, minced
- 2 tsp.s soy sauce
- 1 tsp. oyster sauce
- ½ tsp. kosher salt
- 1 tsp. black pepper

Directions:

1. In the bowl of a stand mixer fitted with the paddle attachment, combine the pork, eggs, green onions,

cilantro, ginger, garlic, soy sauce, oyster sauce, salt, and pepper. Mix on low speed until all of the ingredients are incorporated, 2 to 3 minutes.

2. Form the mixture into 12 meatballs and arrange in a single layer in the Air Fryer basket.

3. Set the Air Fryer to 350°F for 10 minutes. Use a meat thermometer to ensure the meatballs have reached an internal temperature of 145°F.

4. Transfer the meatballs to a bowl and serve.

Nutrition:

Calories 402, Fat 27.91g, Carbs 3.1g, Protein 32.69g

Barbecue Flavored Pork Ribs

Preparation Time: 5 minutes

Cooking Time: 15 minutes

Servings: 6

Ingredients:

- ¼ cup honey, divided
- ¾ cup BBQ sauce
- 2 tbsp. tomato ketchup
- 1 tbsp. Worcestershire sauce
- 1 tbsp. soy sauce
- ½ tsp. garlic powder
- Freshly ground white pepper, to taste
- 1¾ lb. pork ribs

Directions:

1. In a large bowl, mix together 3 tbsp. of honey and remaining ingredients except pork ribs. Refrigerate to marinate for about 20 minutes. Preheat the Air Fryer to 355°F. Place the ribs in an Air Fryer basket.

2. Cook for about 13 minutes. Remove the ribs from the Air Fryer and coat with remaining honey. Serve hot.

Nutrition:

Calories 265, Fat 9.04g, Protein 29.47g, Carbs 15.87g

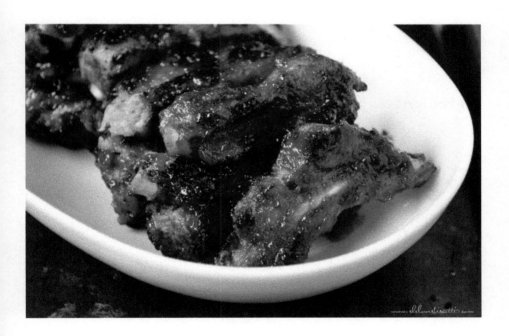

Easy Air Fryer Marinated Pork Tenderloin

Preparation Time: 1 hour & 10 minutes

Cooking Time: 30 minutes

Servings: 4 to 6

Ingredients:

- ¼ cup olive oil
- ¼ cup soy sauce
- ¼ cup freshly squeezed lemon juice
- 1 garlic clove, minced
- 1 tbsp. Dijon mustard
- 1 tsp. salt
- ½ tsp. freshly ground black pepper
- 2 lb. pork tenderloin

Directions:

1. In a large mixing bowl, make the marinade. Mix together the olive oil, soy sauce, lemon juice, minced garlic, Dijon mustard, salt, and pepper. Reserve ¼ cup of the marinade.

2. Place the tenderloin in a large bowl and pour the remaining marinade over the meat. Cover and marinate in the refrigerator for about 1 hour. Place the marinated pork tenderloin into the Air Fryer basket.

3. Set the temperature of your Air Fryer to 400°F. Set the timer and roast for 10 minutes. Using tongs, flip the pork and baste it with half of the reserved marinade. Reset the timer and roast for 10 minutes more.

4. Using tongs, flip the pork, then baste with the remaining marinade.

5. Reset the timer and roast for another 10 minutes, for a total cooking time of 30 minutes.

Nutrition:

Calories 345, Fat 17.35g, Carbs 3.66g, Protein 41.56g

Balsamic Glazed Pork Chops

Preparation Time: 5 minutes

Cooking Time: 50

Servings: 4

Ingredients:

- ¾ cup balsamic vinegar
- 1 ½ tbsp. sugar
- 1 tbsp. butter
- 3 tbsp. olive oil
- 3 tbsp. salt
- 3 pork rib chops

Directions:

1. Place all ingredients in bowl and allow the meat to marinate in the fridge for at least 2 hours. Preheat the Air Fryer to 390°F. Place the grill pan accessory in the Air Fryer.
2. Grill the pork chops for 20 minutes making sure to flip the meat every 10 minutes for even grilling.

Meanwhile, pour the balsamic vinegar on a saucepan and allow to simmer for at least 10 minutes until the sauce thickens. Brush the meat with the glaze before serving.

Nutrition:

Calories 274, Fat 18g, Carbs 7g, Protein17g

Perfect Air Fried Pork Chops

Preparation Time: 5 minutes

Cooking Time: 17 minutes

Servings: 4

Ingredients:

- 3 cups bread crumbs
- ½ cup grated Parmesan cheese
- 2 tbsp. vegetable oil
- 2 tsp.s salt
- 2 tsp.s sweet paprika
- ½ tsp. onion powder
- ¼ tsp. garlic powder
- 6 (½-inch-thick) bone-in pork chops

Directions:

1. Spray the Air Fryer basket with olive oil. In a large resealable bag, combine the bread crumbs, Parmesan cheese, oil, salt, paprika, onion powder, and garlic powder. Seal the bag and shake it a few times in order

for the spices to blend together. Place the pork chops, one by one, in the bag and shake to coat.

2. Place the pork chops in the greased Air Fryer basket in a single layer. Be careful not to overcrowd the basket. Spray the chops generously with olive oil to avoid powdery, uncooked breading.

3. Set the temperature of your Air Fryer to 360°F. Set the timer and roast for 10 minutes.

4. Using tongs, flip the chops. Spray them generously with olive oil. Reset the timer and roast for 7 minutes more.

5. Check that the pork has reached an internal temperature of 145°F. Add cooking time if needed.

Nutrition:

Calories 513, Fat 23g, Carbs 22g, Protein 50g

Rustic Pork Ribs

Preparation Time: 5 minutes

Cooking Time: 15 minutes

Servings: 4

Ingredients:

- 1 rack of pork ribs
- 3 tbsp. dry red wine
- 1 tbsp. soy sauce
- 1/2 tsp. dried thyme
- 1/2 tsp. onion powder
- 1/2 tsp. garlic powder
- 1/2 tsp. ground black pepper
- 1 tsp. smoked salt
- 1 tbsp. cornstarch
- 1/2 tsp. olive oil

Directions:

1. Begin by preheating your Air Fryer to 390°F. Place all ingredients in a mixing bowl and let them marinate for at least 1 hour.

2. Cook the marinated ribs approximately 25 minutes at 390°F. Serve hot.

Nutrition:

Calories 119, Protein 12.26g, Fat 5.61g, Carbs 3.64g

Air Fryer Baby Back Ribs

Preparation Time: 5 minutes

Cooking Time: 25 minutes

Servings: 4

Ingredients:

- 1 rack baby back ribs
- 1 tbsp. garlic powder
- 1 tsp. freshly ground black pepper
- 2 tbsp. salt
- 1 cup barbecue sauce (any type)

Directions:

1. Dry the ribs with a paper towel.
2. Season the ribs with the garlic powder, pepper, and salt. Place the seasoned ribs into the Air Fryer.
3. Set the temperature of your Air Fryer to 400°F. Set the timer and grill for 10 minutes.
4. Using tongs, flip the ribs. Reset the timer and grill for another 10 minutes.

5. Once the ribs are cooked, use a pastry brush to brush on the barbecue sauce, then set the timer and grill for a final 3 to 5 minutes.

Nutrition:

Calories 422, Fat 27g, Carbs 25g, Protein 18g

Parmesan Crusted Pork Chops

Preparation Time: 10 minutes

Cooking Time: 15 minutes

Servings: 8

Ingredients:

- 3 tbsp. grated parmesan cheese
- 1 C. pork rind crumbs
- 2 beaten eggs
- ¼ tsp. chili powder
- ½ tsp. onion powder
- 1 tsp. smoked paprika
- ¼ tsp. pepper
- ½ tsp. salt
- 4-6 thick boneless pork chops

Directions:

1. Ensure your Air Fryer is preheated to 400°F.
2. With pepper and salt, season both sides of pork chops.

3. In a food processor, pulse pork rinds into crumbs. Mix crumbs with other seasonings.
4. Beat eggs and add to another bowl. Dip pork chops into eggs then into pork rind crumb mixture.
5. Spray down Air Fryer with olive oil and add pork chops to the basket. Set temperature to 400°F, and set time to 15 minutes.

Nutrition:

Calories 422, Fat 19g, Carbs 16g, Protein 38g

Crispy Dumplings

Preparation Time: 10 minutes

Cooking Time: 10 minutes

Servings: 8

Ingredients:

- .5 lb. Ground pork
- 1 tbsp. Olive oil
- .5 tsp. each Black pepper and salt
- Half of 1 pkg. Dumpling wrappers

Directions:

1. Set the Air Fryer temperature setting at 390°F.
2. Mix the fixings together. Prepare each dumpling using two tsp.s of the pork mixture.
3. Seal the edges with a portion of water to make the triangle form.
4. Lightly spray the Air Fryer basket using a cooking oil spray as needed. Add the dumplings to air-fry for eight minutes.

5. Serve when they're ready.

Nutrition:

Calories 110, Fat 8.34g, Carbs 0.27g, Protein 8.1g

Pork Joint

Preparation Time: 10 minutes

Cooking Time: 20 minutes

Servings: 10

Ingredients:

- 3 cups Cooked shredded pork tenderloin or chicken
- 2 cups Fat-free shredded mozzarella
- 10 small Flour tortillas
- Lime juice

Directions:

1. Set the Air Fryer at 380°F. Sprinkle the juice over the pork.
2. Microwave five of the tortillas at a time (putting a damp paper towel over them for 10 seconds). Add three oz. of pork and ¼ of a cup of cheese to each tortilla.
3. Tightly roll the tortillas. Line the tortillas onto a greased foil-lined pan.

4. Spray an even coat of cooking oil spray over the tortillas.
5. Air Fry for 7 to 10 minutes or until the tortillas are a golden color, flipping halfway through.

Nutrition:

Calories 334, Fat 6.87g, Protein 32.03g, Carbs 33.92g

Pork Satay

Preparation Time: 15 minutes

Cooking Time: 9-14 minutes

Servings: 4

Ingredients:

- 1 (1-lb.) pork tenderloin, cut into 1½-inch cubes
- ¼ cup minced onion
- garlic cloves, minced
- 1 jalapeño pepper, minced
- tbsp. freshly squeezed lime juice
- tbsp. coconut milk
- tbsp. unsalted peanut butter
- tsp.s curry powder

Directions:

1. In a medium bowl, mix the pork, onion, garlic, jalapeño, lime juice, coconut milk, peanut butter, and

curry powder until well combined. Let stand for 10 minutes at room temperature.

2. With a slotted spoon, remove the pork from the marinade. Reserve the marinade.

3. Thread the pork onto about 8 bamboo (see Tip, here) or metal skewers. Grill for 9 to 14 minutes, brushing once with the reserved marinade, until the pork reaches at least 145°F on a meat thermometer. Discard any remaining marinade. Serve immediately.

Nutrition

Calories 194, Fat 7g, Carbs 7g, Protein 25g

Pork Burgers with Red Cabbage Salad

Preparation Time: 20 minutes

Cooking Time: 7-9 minutes

Servings: 4

Ingredients:

- ½ cup Greek yogurt
- 2 tbsp. low-sodium mustard, divided
- 1 tbsp. lemon juice
- ¼ cup sliced red cabbage
- ¼ cup grated carrots
- 1-lb. lean ground pork
- ½ tsp. paprika
- 1 cup mixed baby lettuce greens
- small tomatoes, sliced
- small low-sodium whole-wheat sandwich buns, cut in half

Directions:

1. In a small bowl, combine the yogurt, 1 tbsp. mustard, lemon juice, cabbage, and carrots; mix and refrigerate.
2. In a medium bowl, combine the pork, remaining 1 tbsp. mustard, and paprika. Form into 8 small patties.
3. Put the sliders into the Air Fryer basket. Grill for 7 to 9 minutes at 370°F, or until the sliders register 165°F as tested with a meat thermometer.
4. Assemble the burgers by placing some of the lettuce greens on a bun bottom. Top with a tomato slice, the - burgers, and the cabbage mixture. Add the bun top and serve immediately.

Nutrition:

Calories 472, Fat 15g, Carbs 15g, Protein 35g

Crispy Mustard Pork Tenderloin

Preparation Time: 10 minutes

Cooking Time: 12-16 minutes

Servings: 4

Ingredients:

- tbsp. low-sodium grainy mustard
- tsp.s olive oil
- ¼ tsp. dry mustard powder
- 1 (1-lb.) pork tenderloin, silver skin and excess fat trimmed and discarded (see Tip, here)
- slices low-sodium whole-wheat bread, crumbled
- ¼ cup ground walnuts
- tbsp. cornstarch

Directions:

1. In a small bowl, stir together the mustard, olive oil, and mustard powder. Spread this mixture over the pork.

36

2. On a plate, mix the bread crumbs, walnuts, and cornstarch. Dip the mustard-coated pork into the crumb mixture to coat.

3. Air fry the pork for 12 to 16 minutes at 370°F, or until it registers at least 145°F on a meat thermometer. Slice to serve.

Nutrition:

Calories 239, Fat 9g, Carbs 15g, Protein 26g

Apple Pork Tenderloin

Preparation Time: 10 minutes

Cooking Time: 14-19 minutes

Servings: 4

Ingredients:

- 1 (1-lb.) pork tenderloin, cut into 4 pieces
- 1 tbsp. apple butter
- 2 tsp.s olive oil
- 2 Granny Smith apples or Jonagold apples, sliced
- 3 celery stalks, sliced
- 1 onion, sliced
- ½ tsp. dried marjoram
- ⅓ cup apple juice

Directions:

1. Rub each piece of pork with the apple butter and olive oil.

2. In a medium metal bowl, mix the pork, apples, celery, onion, marjoram, and apple juice.

3. Place the bowl into the Air Fryer and roast for 14 to 19 minutes at 365°F, or until the pork reaches at least 145°F on a meat thermometer and the apples and vegetables are tender. Stir once during cooking. Serve immediately.

Nutrition:

Calories 21, Fat 5g, Carbs 20g, Protein 24g

Espresso-Grilled Pork Tenderloin

Preparation Time: 15 minutes

Cooking Time: 9-11 minutes

Servings: 4

Ingredients:

- 1 tbsp. packed brown sugar
- 2 tsp.s espresso powder
- 1 tsp. ground paprika
- ½ tsp. dried marjoram
- 1 tbsp. honey
- 1 tbsp. freshly squeezed lemon juice
- 2 tsp.s olive oil
- 1 (1-lb.) pork tenderloin

Directions:

1. In a small bowl, mix the brown sugar, espresso powder, paprika, and marjoram.
2. Stir in the honey, lemon juice, and olive oil until well mixed.
3. Spread the honey mixture over the pork and let stand for 10 minutes at room temperature.
4. Roast the tenderloin in the Air Fryer basket for 9 to 11 minutes at 365°F, or until the pork registers at least 145°F on a meat thermometer. Slice the meat to serve.

Nutrition:

Calories 177, Fat 5g, Carbs 10g, Protein 23g

Pork and Potatoes

Preparation Time: 5 minutes

Cooking Time: 25 minutes

Servings: 4

Ingredients:

- 2 cups creamer potatoes, rinsed and dried
- 2 tsp.s olive oil
- 1 (1-lb.) pork tenderloin, cut into 1-inch cubes
- 1 onion, chopped
- 1 red bell pepper, chopped
- 2 garlic cloves, minced
- ½ tsp. dried oregano
- 2 tbsp. low-sodium chicken broth

Directions:

1. In a medium bowl, toss the potatoes and olive oil to coat.
2. Transfer the potatoes to the Air Fryer basket. Roast for 15 minutes at 380°F.

3. In a medium metal bowl, mix the potatoes, pork, onion, red bell pepper, garlic, and oregano.
4. Drizzle with the chicken broth. Put the bowl in the Air Fryer basket. Roast for about 10 minutes more, shaking the basket once during cooking, until the pork reaches at least 145°F on a meat thermometer and the potatoes are tender. Serve immediately.

Nutrition:

Calories 235, Fat 5g, Carbs 22g, Protein 26g

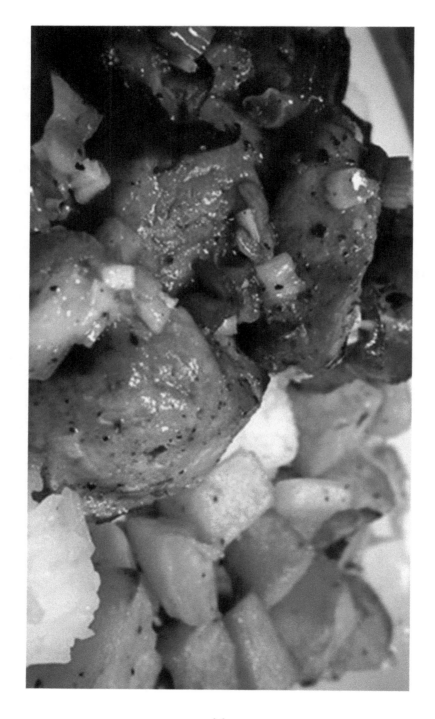

Pork and Fruit Kebabs

Preparation Time: 15 minutes

Cooking Time: 9-12 minutes

Servings: 4

Ingredients:

- ⅓ cup apricot jam
- 2 tbsp. freshly squeezed lemon juice
- 2 tsp.s olive oil
- ½ tsp. dried tarragon
- 1 (1-lb.) pork tenderloin, cut into 1-inch cubes
- 4 plums, pitted and quartered
- 4 small apricots, pitted and halved

Directions:

1. In a large bowl, mix the jam, lemon juice, olive oil, and tarragon.
2. Add the pork and stir to coat. Let stand for 10 minutes at room temperature.

45

3. Alternating the items, thread the pork, plums, and - apricots onto 4 metal skewers that fit into the Air Fryer. Brush with any remaining jam mixture. Discard any remaining marinade.

4. Grill the kebabs in the Air Fryer for 9 to 12 minutes 365°F, or until the pork reaches 145°F on a meat thermometer and the fruit is tender. Serve immediately.

Nutrition:

Calories 256, Fat 5g, Carbs 30g, Protein 24g

Steak and Vegetable Kebabs

Preparation Time: 15 minutes

Cooking Time: 5 to 7 minutes

Servings: 4

Ingredients:

- 2 tbsp. balsamic vinegar
- 2 tsp.s olive oil
- ½ tsp. dried marjoram
- ⅛ tsp. freshly ground black pepper
- ¾ lb. round steak, cut into 1-inch pieces
- 1 red bell pepper, sliced
- 16 button mushrooms
- 1 cup cherry tomatoes

Directions:

1. In a medium bowl, stir together the balsamic vinegar, olive oil, marjoram, and black pepper.

2. Add the steak and stir to coat. Let stand for 10 minutes at room temperature.

3. Alternating items, thread the beef, red bell pepper, mushrooms, and tomatoes onto 8 bamboo (see Tip, here) or metal skewers that fit in the Air Fryer.

4. Grill in the Air Fryer for 5 to 7 minutes at 370°F, or until the beef is browned and reaches at least 145°F on a meat thermometer. Serve immediately.

Nutrition:

Calories 194, Fat 6g, Carbs 7g, Protein 31g

Spicy Grilled Steak

Preparation Time: 7 minutes

Cooking Time: 6 to 9 minutes

Servings: 4

Ingredients:

- 2 tbsp. low-sodium salsa
- 1 tbsp. minced chipotle pepper
- 1 tbsp. apple cider vinegar
- 1 tsp. ground cumin
- ⅛ tsp. freshly ground black pepper
- ⅛ tsp. red pepper flakes
- ¾ lb. sirloin tip steak, cut into 4 pieces and gently pounded to about ⅓ inch thick

Directions:

1. In a small bowl, thoroughly mix the salsa, chipotle pepper, cider vinegar, cumin, black pepper, and red pepper flakes. Rub this mixture into both sides of

49

each steak piece. Let stand for 15 minutes at room temperature.

2. Grill the steaks in the Air Fryer at 365°F, two at a time, for 6 to 9 minutes, or until they reach at least 145°F on a meat thermometer.
3. Remove the steaks to a clean plate and cover with aluminum foil to keep warm. Repeat with the remaining steaks.
4. Slice the steaks thinly against the grain and serve.

Nutrition:

Calories 160, Fat 6g, Carbs 1g, Protein 24g

Greek Vegetable Skillet

Preparation Time: 10 minutes

Cooking Time: 9 to 19 minutes

Servings: 4

Ingredients:

- ½ lb. 96 percent lean ground beef
- 2 medium tomatoes, chopped
- 1 onion, chopped
- 2 garlic cloves, minced
- 2 cups fresh baby spinach
- 2 tbsp. freshly squeezed lemon juice
- ⅓ cup low-sodium beef broth
- 2 tbsp. crumbled low-sodium feta cheese

Directions:

1. In a 6-by-2-inch metal pan, crumble the beef. Cook in the Air Fryer for 3 to 7 minutes at 370°F, stirring

once during cooking, until browned. Drain off any fat or liquid.

2. Add the tomatoes, onion, and garlic to the pan. Air-fry for 4 to 8 minutes more, or until the onion is tender.

3. Add the spinach, lemon juice, and beef broth. Air-fry for 2 to 4 minutes more, or until the spinach is wilted.

4. Sprinkle with the feta cheese and serve immediately

Nutrition:

Calories 97, Fat 1g, Carbs 5g, Protein 15g

Light Herbed Meatballs

Preparation Time: 10 minutes

Cooking Time: 12 to 17 minutes

Servings: 24

Ingredients:

- 1 medium onion, minced
- 2 garlic cloves, minced
- 1 tsp. olive oil
- 1 slice low-sodium whole-wheat bread, crumbled
- 3 tbsp. 1 percent milk
- 1 tsp. dried marjoram
- 1 tsp. dried basil
- 1-lb. 96 percent lean ground beef

Directions:

1. In a 6-by-2-inch pan, combine the onion, garlic, and olive oil. Air-fry for 2 to 4 minutes at 370°F, or until the vegetables are crisp-tender.

2. Transfer the vegetables to a medium bowl, and add the bread crumbs, milk, marjoram, and basil. Mix well.

3. Add the ground beef. With your hands, work the mixture gently but thoroughly until combined. Form the meat mixture into about 24 (1-inch) meatballs.

4. Bake the meatballs, in batches, in the Air Fryer basket for 12 to 17 minutes, or until they reach 160°F on a meat thermometer. Serve immediately.

Nutrition:

Calories 190, Fat 6g, Carbs 8g, Protein 25g

Brown Rice and Beef-Stuffed Bell Peppers

Preparation Time: 10 minutes

Cooking Time: 11 to 16 minutes

Servings: 4

Ingredients:

- 4 medium bell peppers, any colors, rinsed, tops removed
- 1 medium onion, chopped
- ½ cup grated carrot
- 2 tsp.s olive oil
- 2 medium beefsteak tomatoes, chopped
- 1 cup cooked brown rice
- 1 cup chopped cooked low-sodium roast beef
- 1 tsp. dried marjoram

Directions:

1. Remove the stems from the bell pepper tops and chop the tops.
2. In a 6-by-2-inch pan, combine the chopped bell pepper tops, onion, carrot, and olive oil. Cook for 2 to 4 minutes, or until the vegetables are crisp-tender.
3. Transfer the vegetables to a medium bowl. Add the - tomatoes, brown rice, roast beef, and marjoram. Stir to mix.
4. Stuff the vegetable mixture into the bell peppers. Place the bell peppers in the Air Fryer basket. Bake for 11 to 16 minutes at 355°F, or until the peppers are tender and the filling is hot. Serve immediately.

Nutrition:

Calories 206, Fat 6g, Carbs 20g, Protein 18g

Beef and Broccoli

Preparation Time: 10 minutes

Cooking Time: 14 to 18 minutes

Servings: 4

Ingredients:

- 2 tbsp. cornstarch
- ½ cup low-sodium beef broth
- 1 tsp. low-sodium soy sauce
- 12 oz. sirloin strip steak, cut into 1-inch cubes
- 2½ cups broccoli florets
- 1 onion, chopped
- 1 cup sliced cremini mushrooms
- 1 tbsp. grated fresh ginger
- Brown rice, cooked (optional)

Directions:

1. In a medium bowl, stir together the cornstarch, beef broth, and soy sauce.

2. Add the beef and toss to coat. Let stand for 5 minutes at room temperature.

3. With a slotted spoon, transfer the beef from the broth mixture into a medium metal bowl. Reserve the broth.

4. Add the broccoli, onion, mushrooms, and ginger to the beef. Place the bowl into the Air Fryer and cook for 12 to 15 minutes at 370°F, or until the beef reaches at least 145°F on a meat thermometer and the vegetables are tender.

5. Add the reserved broth and cook for 2 to 3 minutes more, or until the sauce boils.

6. Serve immediately over hot cooked brown rice, if desired.

Nutrition:

Calories 240, Fat 6g, Carbs 11g, Protein 19g

Beef and Fruit Stir-Fry

Preparation Time: 15 minutes

Cooking Time: 6 to 11 minutes

Servings: 4

Ingredients:

- 12 oz. sirloin tip steak, thinly sliced
- 1 tbsp. freshly squeezed lime juice
- 1 cup canned mandarin orange segments, drained, juice reserved
- 1 cup canned pineapple chunks, drained, juice reserved
- 1 tsp. low-sodium soy sauce
- 1 tbsp. cornstarch
- 1 tsp. olive oil
- 2 scallions, white and green parts, sliced
- Brown rice, cooked (optional)

Directions:

1. In a medium bowl, mix the steak with the lime juice. Set aside.

2. In a small bowl, thoroughly mix 3 tbsp. of reserved mandarin orange juice, 3 tbsp. of reserved pineapple juice, the soy sauce, and cornstarch.

3. Drain the beef and transfer it to a medium metal bowl, reserving the juice. Stir the reserved juice into the mandarin-pineapple juice mixture. Set aside.

4. Add the olive oil and scallions to the steak. Place the metal bowl in the Air Fryer and cook for 3 to 4 minutes at 365°F, or until the steak is almost cooked, shaking the basket once during cooking.

5. Stir in the mandarin oranges, pineapple, and juice - mixture. Cook for 3 to 7 minutes more, or until the sauce is bubbling and the beef is tender and reaches at least 145°F on a meat thermometer.

6. Stir and serve over hot cooked brown rice, if desired.

Nutrition:

Calories 212, Fat 4g, Carbs 28g, Protein 19g

Garlic Putter Pork Chops

Preparation Time: 10 minutes

Cooking Time: 10 minutes

Servings: 4

Ingredients:

- tsp. parsley
- tsp. grated garlic cloves
- 1 tbsp. coconut oil
- 1 tbsp. coconut butter
- pork chops

Directions:

1. Ensure your Air Fryer is preheated to 350°F.
2. Mix butter, coconut oil, and all seasoning together. Then rub seasoning mixture over all sides of pork chops. Place in foil, seal, and chill for 1 hour.
3. Remove pork chops from foil and place into Air Fryer.

4. Set temperature to 350°F, and set time to 7 minutes. Cook 7 minutes on one side and 8 minutes on the other.

5. Drizzle with olive oil and serve alongside a green salad.

Nutrition:

Calories 526, Fat 23g, Carbs 10g, Protein 41g

Cajun Pork Steaks

Preparation Time: 5 minutes

Cooking Time: 20 minutes

Servings: 6

Ingredients:

- 4-6 pork steaks
- BBQ sauce:
- Cajun seasoning
- 1 tbsp. vinegar
- 1 tsp. low-sodium soy sauce
- ½ C. brown sugar

Directions:

1. Ensure your Air Fryer is preheated to 290°F.
2. Sprinkle pork steaks with Cajun seasoning.
3. Combine remaining ingredients and brush onto steaks. Add coated steaks to Air Fryer.

4. Set temperature to 290°F, and set time to 20 minutes. Cook 15-20 minutes till just browned.

Nutrition:

Calories 209, Fat 11g, Carbs 7g, Protein 28g

Cajun Sweet-Sour Grilled Pork

Preparation Time: 5 minutes

Cooking Time: 12 minutes

Servings: 3

Ingredients:

- ¼ cup brown sugar
- 1/4 cup cider vinegar
- 1-lb pork loin, sliced into 1-inch cubes
- 2 tbsp. Cajun seasoning
- 3 tbsp. brown sugar

Directions:

1. In a shallow dish, mix well pork loin, 3 tbsp. brown sugar, and Cajun seasoning. Toss well to coat. Marinate in the ref for 3 hours.
2. In a medium bowl mix well, brown sugar and vinegar for basting.

3. Thread pork pieces in skewers. Baste with sauce and place on skewer rack in Air Fryer.
4. For 12 minutes, cook on 360°F. Halfway through Cooking Time, turnover skewers and baste with sauce. If needed, cook in batches.
5. Serve and enjoy.

Nutrition:

Calories 428, Fat 16.7g, Carbs 5g, Protein 39g

Pork Loin with Potatoes

Preparation Time: 10 minutes

Cooking Time: 25 minutes

Servings: 2

Ingredients:

- 2 lb. pork loin
- large red potatoes, chopped
- ½ tsp. garlic powder
- ½ tsp. red pepper flakes, crushed
- Salt and black pepper, to taste

Directions:

1. In a large bowl, put all of the ingredients together except glaze and toss to coat well. Preheat the Air Fryer to 325°F. Place the loin in the Air Fryer basket.
2. Arrange the potatoes around pork loin.
3. Cook for about 25 minutes.

Nutrition:

   Calories 260, Fat 8g, Carbs 27g, Protein 21g

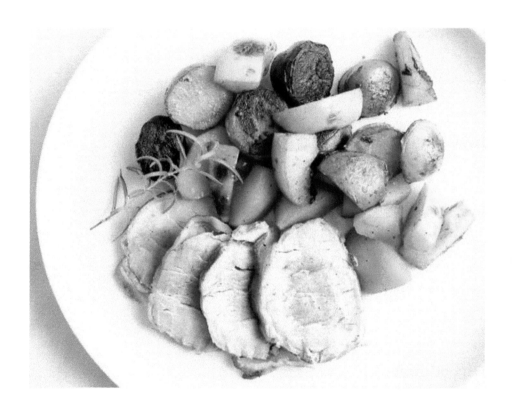

Roasted Char Siew (Pork Butt)

Preparation Time: 10 minutes

Cooking Time: 25 minutes

Servings: 4

Ingredients:

- 1 strip of pork shoulder butt with a good amount of fat marbling
- Marinade:
  a. 1 tsp. sesame oil
  b. tbsp. raw honey
  c. 1 tsp. light soy sauce
  d. 1 tbsp. rose wine

Directions:

1. Mix all of the marinade ingredients together and put it to a Ziploc bag. Place pork in bag, making sure all sections of pork strip are engulfed in the marinade. Chill 3-24 hours.

2. Take out the strip 30 minutes before planning to cook and preheat your Air Fryer to 350°F.
3. Place foil on small pan and brush with olive oil. Place marinated pork strip onto prepared pan.
4. Set temperature to 350°F, and set time to 20 minutes. Roast 20 minutes.
5. Glaze with marinade every 5-10 minutes.
6. Remove strip and leave to cool a few minutes before slicing.

Nutrition:

Calories 289, Fat 13g, Carbs 6g, Protein33g

Asian Pork Chops

Preparation Time: 2 hours and 10 minutes
Cooking Time: 15 minutes
Servings: 2

Ingredients:

- 1/2 cup hoisin sauce
- tbsp. cider vinegar
- 1 tbsp. Asian sweet chili sauce
- (1/2-inch-thick) boneless pork chops
- salt and pepper

Directions:

1. Stir together hoisin, chili sauce, and vinegar in a large mixing bowl. Separate a quarter cup of this mixture, then add pork chops to the bowl and let it sit in the fridge for 2 hours. Take out the pork chops and place them on a plate. Sprinkle each side of the pork chop evenly with salt and pepper.
2. Cook at 360°For 14 minutes, flipping half way through. Brush with reserved marinade and serve.

Nutrition: Calories 338, Fat 21g, Carbs 28g, Protein 19g

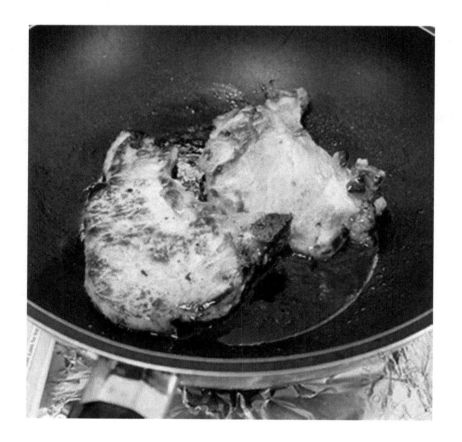

Marinated Pork Chops

Preparation Time: 10 minutes

Cooking Time: 30 minutes

Servings: 2

Ingredients:

- pork chops, boneless
- 1 tsp. garlic powder
- ½ cup flour
- 1 cup buttermilk
- Salt and pepper

Directions:

1. Add pork chops and buttermilk in a zip-lock bag. Seal the bag and set aside in the refrigerator overnight.
2. In another zip-lock bag add flour, garlic powder, pepper, and salt.
3. Remove marinated pork chops from buttermilk and add in flour mixture and shake until well coated.
4. Preheat the Air Fryer oven to 380°F.

5. Spray Air Fryer tray with cooking spray.
6. Arrange pork chops on a tray and Air Fryer for 28-30 minutes. Turn pork chops after 18 minutes.
7. Serve and enjoy.

Nutrition:

Calories 424, Fat 21.3g, Carbs 30.8g, Protein 25.5g

Steak with Cheese Butter

Preparation Time: 10 minutes

Cooking Time: 8-10 minutes

Servings: 2

Ingredients:

- 2 rib-eye steaks
- tsp. garlic powder
- 1/2 tbsp. blue cheese butter
- 1 tsp. pepper
- tsp. kosher salt

Directions:

1. Preheat the Air Fryer to 400°F.
2. Mix together garlic powder, pepper, and salt and rub over the steaks.
3. Spray Air Fryer basket with cooking spray.

4. Put the steak in the Air Fryer basket and cook for 4-5 minutes on each side.
5. Top with blue butter cheese.
6. Serve and enjoy.

Nutrition:

Calories 830, Fat 60g, Carbs 3g, Protein 70g

Madeira Beef

Preparation Time: 5 minutes

Cooking Time: 25 minutes

Servings: 6

Ingredients:

- 1 cup Madeira
- 1 and ½ lb. beef meat, cubed
- Salt and black pepper to the taste
- 1 yellow onion, thinly sliced
- 1 chili pepper, sliced

Directions:

1. Put the reversible rack in the Air Fryer, add the baking pan inside and mix all the ingredients in it.
2. Cook on Baking mode at 380°F for 25 minutes, divide the mix into bowls and serve.

Nutrition:

Calories 295, Fat 16, Carbs 20, Protein 15

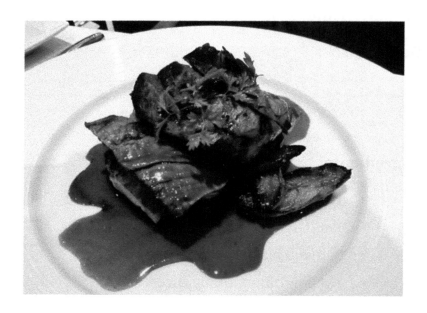

Creamy Pork and Zucchinis

Preparation Time: 5 minutes

Cooking Time: 25 minutes

Servings: 4

Ingredients:

- 1 and ½ lb. pork stew meat, cubed
- 1 cup tomato sauce
- 1 tbsp. olive oil
- 2 zucchinis, sliced
- Salt and black pepper to the taste

Directions:

1. Put the reversible rack in the Air Fryer, add the baking pan inside and mix all the ingredients in it.
2. Cook on Baking mode at 380°F, divide the mix into bowls and serve.

Nutrition: Calories 284, Fat 12, Carbs 17, Protein 12

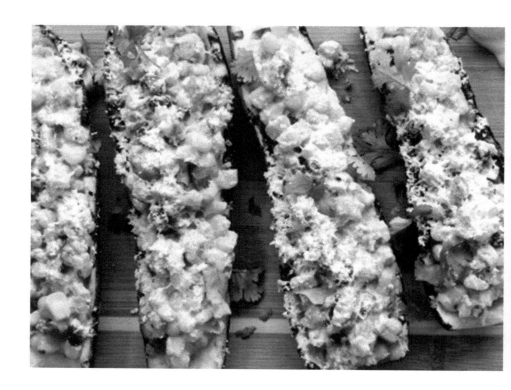

Bullet-proof Beef Roast

Preparation Time: 2 hours

Cooking Time: 2 hours and 5 minutes

Servings: 2

Ingredients:

- 1 cup of organic beef
- tbsp. olive oil
- 1 lb. beef round roast
- Salt and pepper, to taste

Directions:

1. Place all of the ingredients in a resealable bag and let it marinate in the fridge for about two hours.
2. Fix the temperature to 400°F and preheat the Air Fryer for 5 minutes.
3. Place the ingredients in the Ziploc bag in a baking tray that will fit the Air Fryer.
4. Let it cook for 2 hours at a temperature of 400°F.

5. Serve while it is warm.

Nutrition:

Calories 280, Fat 15g, Carbs 13g, Protein 26g

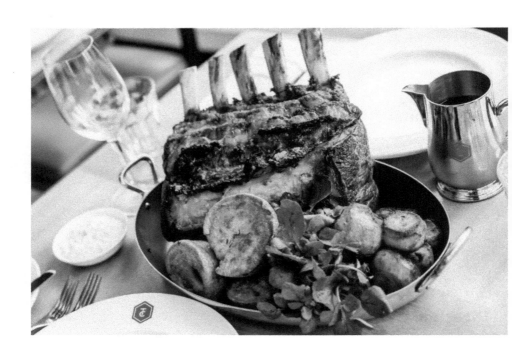

Lamb Burgers

Preparation Time: 15 minutes

Cooking Time: 8 minutes

Servings: 6

Ingredients:

- 2 lb. ground lamb
- 1 tbsp. onion powder
- Salt and ground black pepper, as required

Directions:

1. In a bowl, add all the ingredients and mix well.
2. Make 6 equal-sized patties from the mixture. Arrange the patties onto a cooking tray.
3. Arrange the drip pan in the bottom of the Air Fryer.
4. Air fry for 8 minutes at 360°F and turn the burgers after 4 minutes
5. When cooking time is complete, remove the tray from Air Fryer and serve hot.

Nutrition:

Calories 285, Carbs 0.9g, Fat 11.1g, Protein 42.6g

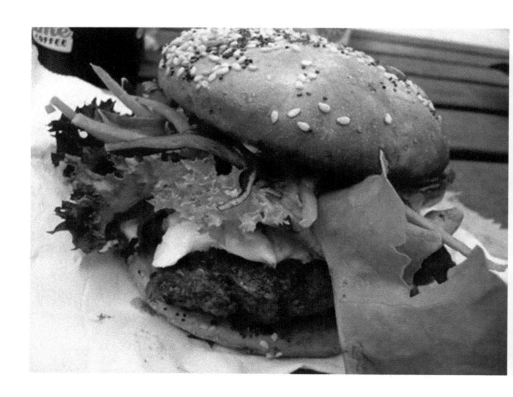

FISH AND SEAFOOD

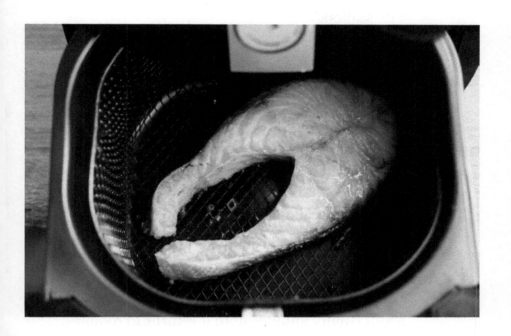

Lemon Butter Scallops

Preparation Time: 1 hour 5 minutes

Cooking Time: 10 minutes

Servings: 4

Ingredients:

- 1 lemon
- 1 lb. scallops
- ½ cup butter
- ¼ cup parsley, chopped

Directions:

1. Juice the lemon into a Ziploc bag.
2. Wash your scallops, dry them, and season to taste. Put them in the bag with the lemon juice. Refrigerate for an hour.
3. Remove the bag from the refrigerator and leave for about twenty minutes until it returns to room temperature. Transfer the scallops into a foil pan that is small enough to be placed inside the fryer.
4. Pre-heat the fryer at 400°F and put the rack inside.
5. Place the foil pan on the rack, and cook for five minutes.
6. In the meantime, melt the butter in a saucepan over a medium heat. Zest the lemon over the saucepan, then add in the chopped parsley. Mix well.
7. Take care when removing the pan from the fryer. Transfer the contents to a plate and drizzle with the lemon-butter mixture. Serve hot.

Nutrition:

Calories 412
Fat 17g
Carbs 18g
Protein 26g

Cheesy Lemon Halibut

Preparation Time: 5 minutes

Cooking Time: 10 minutes

Servings: 4

Ingredients:

- 1 lb. halibut fillet
- ½ cup butter
- 2 ½ tbsp. mayonnaise
- 2 ½ tbsp. lemon juice
- ¾ cup parmesan cheese, grated

Directions:

1. Pre-heat your fryer at 375°F.
2. Spritz the halibut fillets with cooking spray and season as desired.
3. Put the halibut in the fryer and cook for twelve minutes.

4. In the meantime, combine the butter, mayonnaise, and lemon juice in a bowl with a hand mixer. Ensure a creamy texture is achieved.
5. Stir in the grated parmesan.
6. When the halibut is ready, open the drawer and spread the butter over the fish with a butter knife. Let it cook for a couple more minutes, then serve hot.

Nutrition:

Calories 354
Fat 21g
Carbs 23g
Protein 19g

Spicy Mackerel

Preparation Time: 5 minutes

Cooking Time: 10 minutes

Servings: 4

Ingredients:

- 2 mackerel fillets
- 2 tbsp. red chili flakes
- 2 tsp. garlic, minced
- 1 tsp. lemon juice

Directions:

1. Season the mackerel fillets with the red pepper flakes, minced garlic, and a drizzle of lemon juice. Allow to sit for five minutes.
2. Preheat your fryer at 350°F.
3. Cook the mackerel for five minutes, before opening the drawer, flipping the fillets, and allowing to cook on the other side for another five minutes.

4. Plate the fillets, making sure to spoon any remaining juice over them before serving.

Nutrition:

Calories 393

Fat 12g

Carbs 13g

Protein 35g

Thyme Scallops

Preparation Time: 5 minutes

Cooking Time: 10 minutes

Servings: 4

Ingredients:

- 1 lb. scallops
- Salt and pepper
- ½ tbsp. butter
- ½ cup thyme, chopped

Directions:

1. Wash the scallops and dry them completely. Season with pepper and salt, then set aside while you prepare the pan.
2. Grease a foil pan in several spots with the butter and cover the bottom with the thyme. Place the scallops on top.
3. Pre-heat the fryer at 400°F and set the rack inside.

4. Place the foil pan on the rack and allow to cook for seven minutes.

5. Take care when removing the pan from the fryer and transfer the scallops to a serving dish. Spoon any remaining butter in the pan over the fish and enjoy.

Nutrition:

Calories 454

Fat 18g

Carbs 27g

Protein 34g

Chinese Style Cod

Preparation Time: 5 minutes

Cooking Time: 10 minutes

Servings: 2

Ingredients:

- 2 medium cod fillets; boneless
- 1 tbsp. light soy sauce
- 1/2 tsp. ginger; grated
- 1 tsp. peanuts; crushed
- 2 tsp. garlic powder

Directions:

1. Put fish fillets in a heat proof dish that fits your Air Fryer, add garlic powder, soy sauce and ginger; toss well, put in your Air Fryer and cook at 350°F, for 10 minutes.
2. Divide fish on plates, sprinkle peanuts on top and serve.

Nutrition:

Calories 254

Fat 10g

Carbs 14g

Protein 23g

Mustard Salmon Recipe

Preparation Time: 5 minutes

Cooking Time: 10 minutes

Servings: 4

Ingredients:

- 1 big salmon fillet; boneless
- 2 tbsp. mustard
- 1 tbsp. coconut oil
- 1 tbsp. maple extract
- Salt and black pepper to the taste

Directions:

1. In a bowl; mix maple extract with mustard, whisk well, season salmon with salt and pepper and brush salmon with this mix.
2. Spray some cooking spray over fish; place in your Air Fryer and cook at 370°F, for 10 minutes; flipping halfway. Serve with a tasty side salad.

Nutrition:

Calories 300

Fat 7g

Carbs 16g

Protein 20g

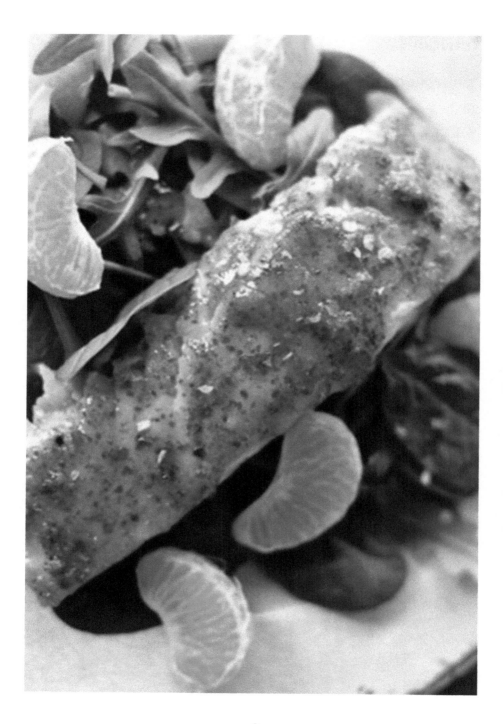

Salmon and Orange Marmalade Recipe

Preparation Time: 5 minutes

Cooking Time: 20 minutes

Servings: 4

Ingredients:

- 1 lb. wild salmon; skinless, boneless and cubed
- 1/4 cup orange juice
- 1/3 cup orange marmalade
- 1/4 cup balsamic vinegar
- A pinch of salt and black pepper

Directions:

1. Heat up a pot with the vinegar over medium heat; add marmalade and orange juice; stir, bring to a simmer, cook for 1 minute and take off heat.
2. Thread salmon cubes on skewers, season with salt and black pepper, brush them with half of the orange marmalade mix, arrange in your Air Fryer's basket

and cook at 360°F, for 3 minutes on each side. Brush skewers with the rest of the vinegar mix; divide among plates and serve right away with a side salad.

Nutrition:

Calories 240

Fat 9g

Carbs 14g

Protein 10g

Tilapia & Chives Sauce

Preparation Time: 5 minutes

Cooking Time: 10 minutes

Servings: 4

Ingredients:

- 4 medium tilapia fillets
- 2 tsp. honey
- Juice from 1 lemon
- 2 tbsp. chives; chopped
- Salt and black pepper to the taste

Directions:

1. Flavor fish with salt and pepper, spray with cooking spray, place in preheated Air Fryer 350°F and cook for 8 minutes; flipping halfway.
2. Meanwhile; in a bowl, mix honey, salt, pepper, chives and lemon juice and whisk really well. Divide Air Fryer fish on plates, drizzle yogurt sauce all over and serve right away.

Nutrition:

Calories 261g

Fat 8g

Carbs 24g

Protein 21g

Buttery Shrimp Skewers

Preparation Time: 5 minutes

Cooking Time: 10 minutes

Servings: 4

Ingredients:

- 8 shrimps; peeled and deveined
- 8 green bell pepper slices
- 1 tbsp. butter; melted
- 4 garlic cloves; minced
- Salt and black pepper to the taste

Directions:

1. In a bowl; mix shrimp with garlic, butter, salt, pepper and bell pepper slices; toss to coat and leave aside for 10 minutes.
2. Arrange 2 shrimp and 2 bell pepper slices on a skewer and repeat with the rest of the shrimp and bell pepper pieces.

3. Place them all in your Air Fryer's basket and cook at 360°F for 6 minutes. Divide among plates and serve right away.

Nutrition:

Calories 140
Fat 1g
Carbs 15g
Protein 7g

Marinated Salmon Recipe

Preparation Time: 1 hour and 5 minutes

Cooking Time: 30 minutes

Servings: 4

Ingredients:

- 1 whole salmon
- 1 tbsp. tarragon; chopped
- 1 tbsp. garlic; minced
- Juice from 2 lemons
- A pinch of salt and black pepper

Directions:

1. In a large fish, mix fish with salt, pepper and lemon juice; toss well and keep in the fridge for 1 hour.
2. Stuff salmon with garlic and place in your Air Fryer's basket and cook at 320°F for 25 minutes. Divide among plates and serve with a tasty coleslaw on the side.

Nutrition:

Calories 300

Fat 8g

Carbs 19g

Protein 27g

Tasty Grilled Red Mullet

Preparation Time: 5 minutes

Cooking Time: 10 minutes

Servings: 8

Ingredients:

- 8 whole red mullets, gutted and scales removed
- Salt and pepper to taste
- Juice from 1 lemon
- 1 tbsp. olive oil

Directions:

1. Preheat the Air Fryer at 390°F.
2. Place the grill pan attachment in the Air Fryer.
3. Season the red mullet with salt, pepper, and lemon juice.
4. Brush with olive oil.
5. Grill for 15 minutes.

Nutrition:

Calories 152

Fat 6.2g

Carbs 0.9g

Protein 23.1g

Garlicky-Grilled Turbot

Preparation Time: 5 minutes

Cooking Time: 20 minutes

Servings: 2

Ingredients:

- 2 whole turbot, scaled and head removed
- Salt and pepper to taste
- 1 clove of garlic, minced
- ½ cup chopped celery leaves
- 2 tbsp. olive oil

Directions:

1. Preheat the Air Fryer at 390°F.
2. Place the grill pan attachment in the Air Fryer.
3. Flavor the turbot with salt, pepper, garlic, and celery leaves.
4. Brush with oil.
5. Cook in the grill pan for 20 minutes until the fish becomes flaky.

Nutrition:

Calories 269

Fat 25.6g

Carbs 3.3g

Protein 66.2g

Lightning Source UK Ltd.
Milton Keynes UK
UKHW020640220621
385951UK00004B/76